TABLE OF CONTENTS

Introduction

I could drop weight fairly easily in my 20s. Calorie reduction, adding fiber, water and a little more exercise was all I had to do. In my 30s, it got a little harder. So, I learned about lowering fat and carbohydrate intake. That worked well for about 10 years.

Then, around the age of 45 or so, peri-menopause was in full swing and my metabolism had retired! *I'd have 900 to 1200 calories of protein and complex carbs, with just 5 – 10 grams of fat a day for weeks on end* **and NOT lose one pound.** Exercise would keep me toned up, but it would not help me lose weight.

Through research and trial and error over several years, I have learned that **weight loss can be achieved** in simple, palatable steps, EVEN as you get older and EVEN when other weight loss techniques and programs no longer or never have worked!

The Steps

There are only **ten** steps in the Weight Loss In Steps program. Each step is important. For some people, certain steps are going to be more important than others.

The **Weight Loss In Steps** program is extremely **flexible**. You decide when you are going to take an additional step.

There is nothing that says you must take all ten steps as quickly as possible. Although, I have no doubt some of you will. Some of you may want to do the opposite, go very slowly. Fine! One new step a week is a step! Most of you will end up somewhere in the middle, taking on a few new steps at once. Each of these choices will work. Progress is progress!

Once you take a specific step, **you need to fully incorporate it**. This means from that day forward, you will continue to take (follow) that step. This allows you to progress and it creates momentum. Thankfully, there are only 10 steps! Note: You don't have to take these steps in order.

Is there an easy way to know if you might be taking on too few or many steps at once? Yes, use this simple test to help you determine the speed that is right for you:

Ask yourself, "*How do I feel about the steps that I have taken so far?*"

If your response is, "*Great!* *I'm looking forward to taking another new step*", you should continue at the same rate.

If your response is, "*OK. But, I would like to do more at once.*", you should <u>increase</u> your rate for taking a new step.

If your response is, "*I'm overwhelmed! And I dread more changes.*", you should <u>slow</u> your rate for taking a new step.

You **must avoid** being **overwhelmed and feeling dread**. If it happens it means that you are doing way too much at once.

Why do we need to pay attention to this red flag? If/when you hit this point, you **exponentially** increase the likelihood of <u>not keeping up the routine and using this system.</u> If this happens to you, it doesn't matter how fast you got to where you are and how much progress you've made up to that point. You are overwhelmed and could reject the whole thing any second. At which point, you'd begin to undo your progress fairly rapidly.

You've got to keep this system palatable by taking on only what you are OK with taking on so that you can be neutral or better about the notion of continuing with the system for the foreseeable future.

STEP 1 Reduce Your Salt

Many people never realize that it's the **high salt** that in their diet that is causing them to **hold onto** a lot of their **weight**.

Some can lose weight during their twenties, thirties and even most of their forties without paying much attention to salt. When you notice your ankles are swelling towards the end of the day and you can't get rings off your fingers at night, you at least begin to realize something is going on.

Doctors may tell you to stop the salt intake cold turkey. Good luck. **It's in everything**. And I mean everything. Low hanging fruit here includes not using the salt shaker, not eating any deli meats and most canned soup. But that may not be enough for a good number of you. For you, it's necessary to count the milligrams of salt you are ingesting daily. And, you'll watch for what accumulated total amount triggers the water retention.

I have become so sensitive to salt that I really have to avoid it. I have tried the Morton's Salt Substitute. Try it. It's not that great tasting. But it does resemble salt (it is Potassium). Depending on what you use it for, you may find it is fine.

I prefer **Bernard Jensen's Vegetable Seasoning**. I've been using it for many years. And although its ingredients have changed a bit over time, it still has a ton of vegetables in it. And it tastes really delicious. Whether it is put on pasta, vegetables, eggs or fish, this seasoning makes the food taste good. And, I am fussy about flavors! With any luck, you will feel as I do, and you will not miss salt when you use this seasoning. In other words: This concoction, for me, has been a **silver bullet** for quickly and happily reducing your salt intake.

STEP 2 Halve Your Carbs

You need to **at least** halve your carbs. This is a very simple and powerful step, especially for men! And, I am convinced that while I was still in my twenties, this worked great for me as well.

What is **essential** here is that you are completely **honest** about what you normally would have and follow through with cutting those carbs in half. Otherwise you are playing games and wasting your time because you will not be successful.

This rule holds true for ALL carbs. This includes **alcohol**. Now, if you think that by having some alcohol you will forget the rule or you may become apt to no longer care about the rule for the rest of the day, don't have any alcohol!

There are women that will have to reduce their carbs by more (like 75%). But 50% is a great first step. And, a good number of you may find that 50% is enough.

One neat thing is, you can still make sandwiches. You just need to be creative. This grilled turkey patty with cucumber is scrumptious with a little mustard/dill vinegar sauce. In the really warm weather, I get rid of the bread entirely and have the cucumber on the top and bottom.

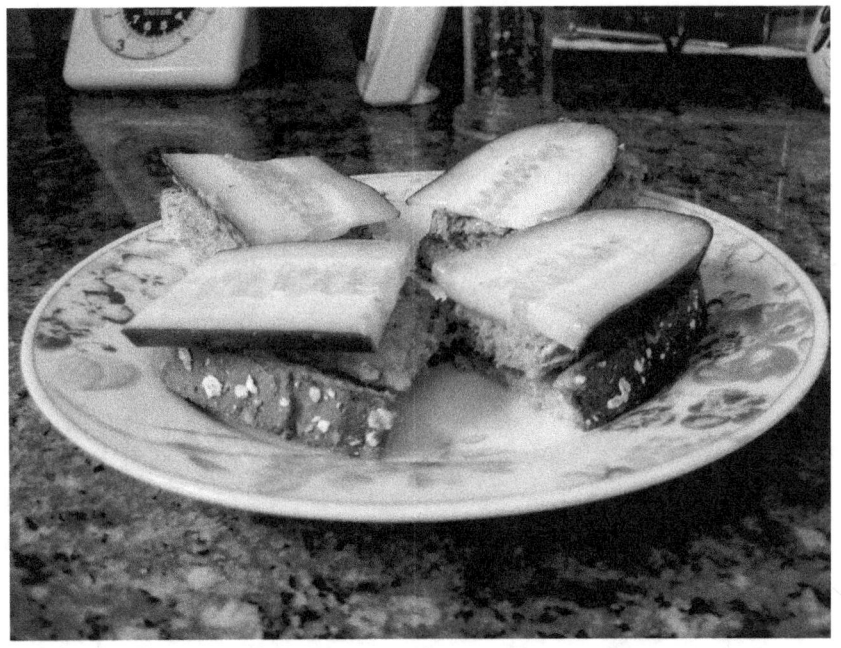

Grilled Turkey Patty With Cucumber Sandwich

STEP 3 Eat These Vegetables

A well known Traditional Chinese Medicine practitioner in Boston treated me a few years ago. Aside from the herbs he prescribed, he told me to eat these two vegetables on a very regular basis. Daily would be best. They are raw, very fresh and juicy celery and cucumber.

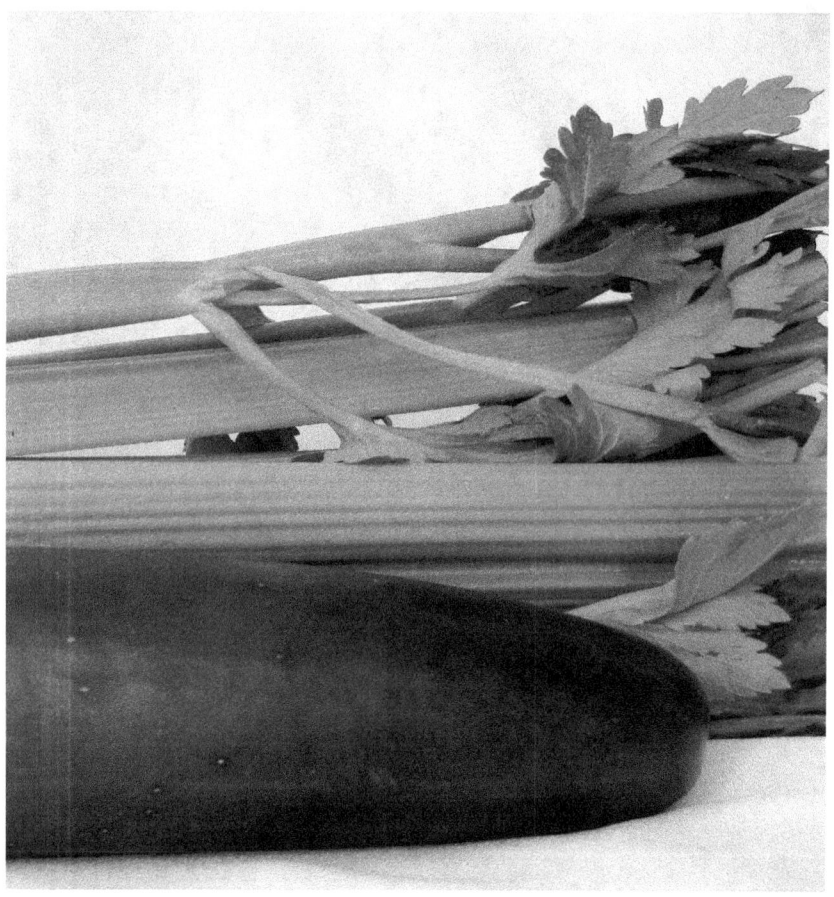

Very Fresh and Juicy Celery and Cucumber

There is something very special about these two vegetables. I feel so much better when I eat them. They really seem to **help your body help itself.**

Celery in particular, has a number of amazing health benefits:

Blood Ph: The minerals in celery juice regulate the body's blood pH, neutralizing acidity.

Blood Pressure: *Phtalides, a compound,* helps relax the muscle around arteries, dilating the vessels and allowing blood to flow normally.

Body Fluid: The sodium and potassium in the celery helps to regulate body fluid and stimulate urine production. This helps to eliminate excessive body fluid.

Body Temperature: Drinking celery juice two or three times a day, between meals can help normalize body temperature. This is especially useful during heat waves.

Cholesterol: The juice has been shown to considerably lower total cholesterol and LDL (bad) cholesterol.

Disease: Celery contains a minimum of eight sets of anti-cancer compounds. These include *acetylenics* which have been shown to stop the growth of tumor cells. *Coumarins* which help prevent free radicals from damaging cells. And, *Phenolic acids:* These block the action of prostaglandins that promote the growth of tumor cells.

Electrolytes: Celery juice is a very good post-workout beverage since it can replace lost electrolytes and rehydrates the body with minerals.

Inflammation: The *polyacetylene* in celery provides remarkable relief for all inflammation like rheumatoid arthritis, osteoarthritis, bronchitis, gout, and asthma

Kidney Function: Celery promotes healthy and normal kidney function by improving elimination of toxins from the body. Additionally, it prevents formation of kidney stones.

Regularity: The laxative effect of celery helps to relieve constipation. It also helps calm nerves which have been overworked by OTC laxatives.

Aside from eating cucumber and celery on their own, you can make a smoothie that is predominantly made out of these ingredients. Sounds weird? Once you try this drink, you will see that it isn't. The recipe has been tweaked to have this be a very healthy, delicious and satisfying beverage.

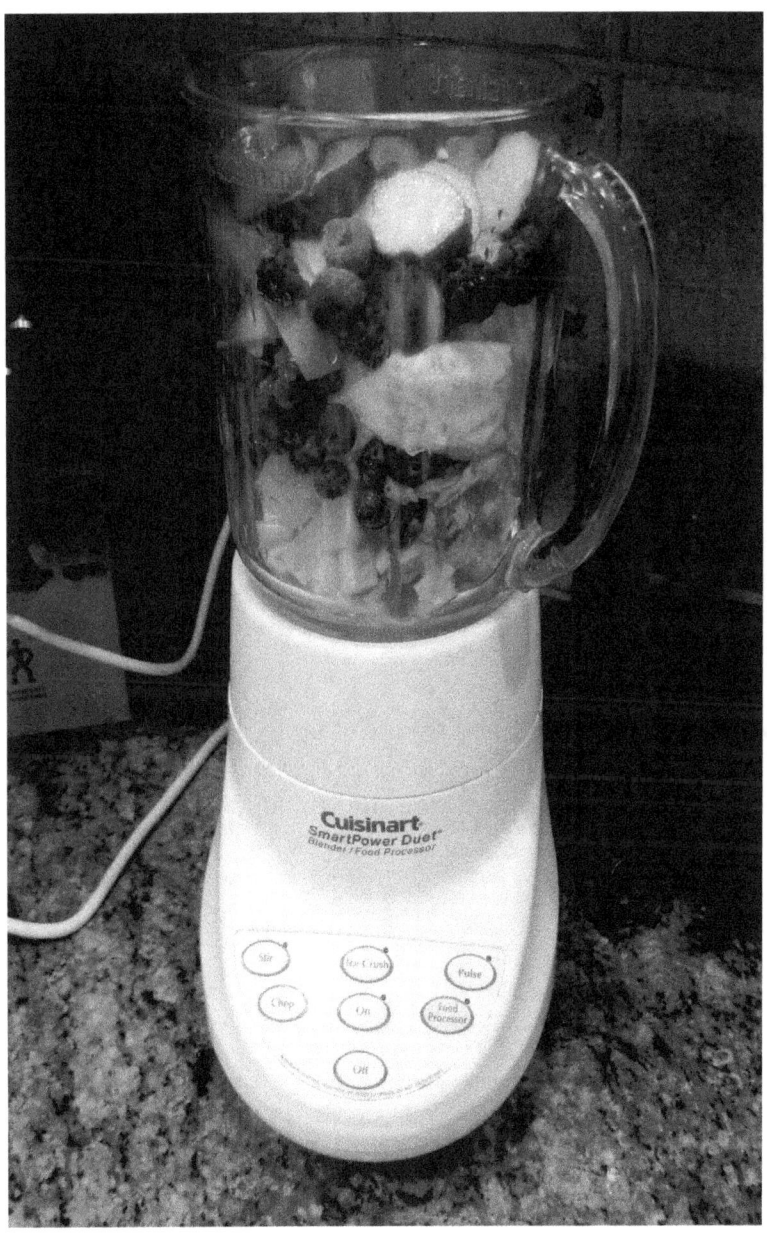

Weight Loss In Steps Smoothie Ingredients

Weight Loss In Steps Smoothie cont'd

2 large stalks of fresh celery
2 small (dill pickle size) or 1/2 medium fresh cucumbers
1/3 cup low sodium/no salt added, 1 % fat cottage cheese (get closest you can find)
1 tsp cold pressed flax seed oil (the kind that is refrigerated at the market)
1/2 small preferably frozen banana
1/2 lemon peeled and deseeded
1 small or 1/2 large Granny Smith apple cored
1/3 cup preferably frozen raspberries and blueberries
1/3 cup spring/bottled water
6 to 12 drops (or more to taste) of Stevia flavored sweetener (lemon, orange, vanilla, berry flavors work great)

Directions

Chop the fresh vegetables and fruit. Cut up frozen banana.

Put all ingredients in blender. Mix until smooth. Pour into 2+ cup glass. Enjoy!

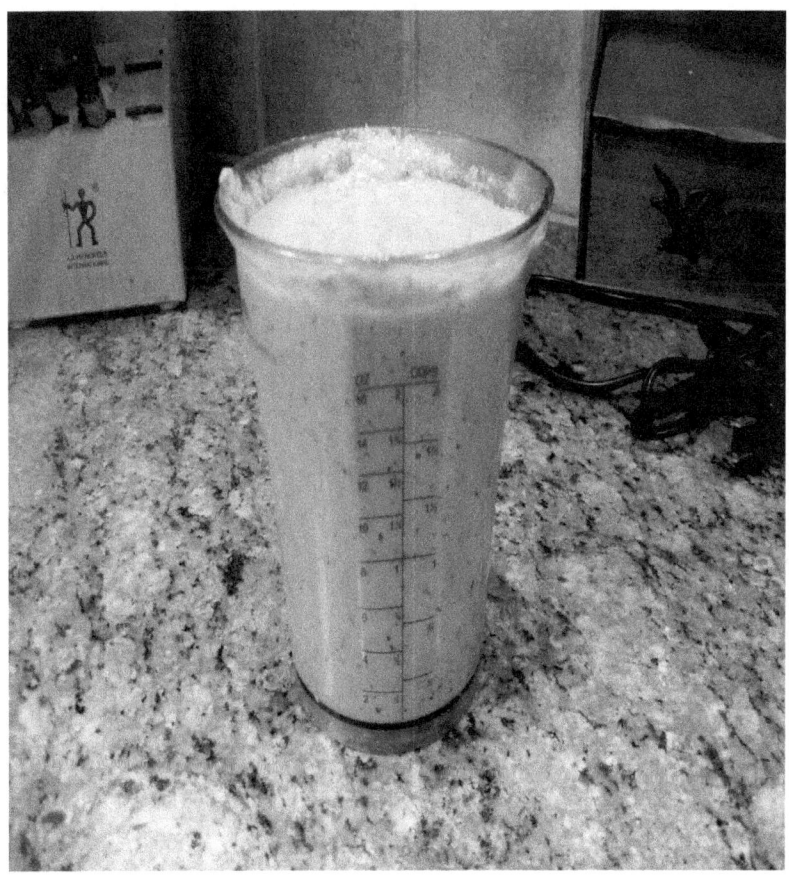

Weight Loss In Steps Smoothie

In the summer I work up to at least one of these a day, often two. And once a week I will have this smoothie for my main three meals. You will not feel deprived or hungry. And, you can almost feel your body thanking you for giving it nutritious food it can really use.

STEP 4 Eat These Fruits

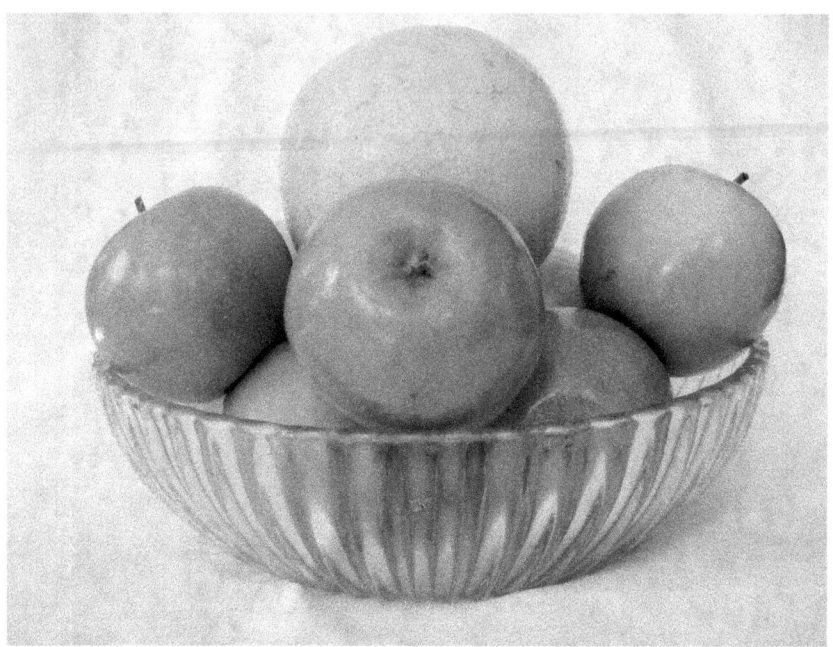

White Grapefruit and Granny Smith Apples

You need to begin to focus on having these two fruits: **White Grapefruit** and **Granny Smith apples**.

They have less sugar and yet still satisfy that need for something sweet now and again. They also contain a good amount of fiber. White Grapefruit additionally has a decent amount of Vitamin C, Potassium, Beta Carotene & Lycopene.

STEP 5 Drink Enough Water

If you do everything else right and you are dehydrated, you **will not** lose weight efficiently. Many of us are dehydrated and don't even know it.

Try your best to work up to **eight 8 oz glasses of water a day**. I find that my body seems to want water in the middle of the night. That counts!

Certainly when you feel thirsty through out the day, make sure you have water on hand. Your body really **needs water** when you actually notice you are **thirsty**. It is generally best to try to drink water in fairly even amounts over the course of 24 hours.

STEP 6 Reduce or Eliminate Certain Sweeteners

You need to significantly cut back on your use of sugar, if you ingest a lot of it.   Sugar spikes your insulin and glucose levels. This causes your body to **more easily store fat**. It also tends to **lead to overeating**. Additionally it can undermine to your heart health, as it can raise blood pressure, triglycerides and bad cholesterol.

You need to eliminate certain low-cal sugar substitutes such as: Sweet n Low, Equal and Splenda from your diet as the safety of their chemical composition has been called into question.

The good news is there is a newer sweetener that appears to be absolutely fine (*at least at this writing*) and really works fantastically well. It's called **Stevia**. Truvia is an excellent brand as it dissolves like sugar and is not bitter at all.

Stevia, unfortunately is expensive. Hopefully, the price will come down as supplies increase.

STEP 7 Evaluate Preserved Foods

There are several problems with these. The biggest one is the **hidden** salt. Even the enormously popular diet plans' meals on TV have very high amounts of salt in them. You need to **stay away from** most if not all of them. This includes: deli meats, canned soups and vegetables, standard soup bouillon, and all prepackaged microwavable meals. And, **stick to fresh or frozen vegetables.** An exception here is when you've been able to find a low or no sodium vegetable in a can or box.

STEP 8 Reduce/Eliminate Dairy Consumption and Avoid Bad Fats

Dairy is mucous forming and is hard on many systems. Protein and calcium are two things that people like to get from dairy. If you insist on keeping some of it, keep % of fat and sodium very low and digestibility of the cheese, high (*ricotta, cottage cheese, mozzarella are easier to digest*).

Having anything deep fried will sabotage this plan. Reduce your fat intake significantly. And the fat that you do have daily should be in the form of high quality **cold pressed olive oil or flax seed oil.**

STEP 9 Give Yourself Satisfying Yet Smart Snacks

Two times a day, you need to have a **snack**. So, every couple hours you will be eating. This will cause your metabolism speed up, which is so critical as we get older.

What is also critical here is **keeping the right snacks** on hand (*and ideally, not having the wrong ones available*).

Why? When you need a snack, you are often hungry and maybe even a little fussy because you are hungry. If you don't have the right snacks on hand that also taste good, you are apt to select something that will not be a good decision.

Set yourself up for success by having good, appropriate snacks on hand (*and in some cases, pre-portion them so that you can simply grab them when needed*).

Some of the snacks that serve me well are:

Blanched almonds 5 to 10

Almond/rice crisp crackers- 10 – 20

Mission Figs- 1-2 fresh/dried

Carrots and celery 1 cup portions- cut up and put in snack plastic bags (and kept in the refrigerator) with 1/8 to 1/4 cup of humus

Granny Smith apple- 1 small or ½ med

White Grapefruit- ½ medium or ¼ large

Whey protein- 10 grams (see Protein dial below)

Structure around snacking is one factor that helps those expensive televised weight loss programs to work. These programs actually create a great deal of structure around the snacks you have daily. For example, you have to have "their" crisps and "their" wafers, etc. It is necessary to have structure around snacking. But it **doesn't have to** be quite as structured as they might lead you to believe, in order for you to be successful.

Additionally, The Weight Loss In Steps program requires snacks with certain, high quality characteristics. Other programs allow snacks with problematic ingredients. For example, **the salt they add** can be a real problem. This was the case for me once I was in my early 40s. .

STEP 10 Walk!

You can start with as little as **5 minutes** a day if you wish. There is still some benefit. Work up to at least a **30 minute** brisk walk **3 to 7 days** a week. I'd like to see you eventually get to about an hour. Bring water to drink.

I personally feel that an interesting walk helps you to stick with it. One of my favorite walks was done at lunch when I was working in Cambridge, MA. We were at 1 Main St. You'd begin by walking along the Charles River on Memorial Drive and then cross over the river via the Mass Ave Bridge. Then, you'd continue along the river towards the Longfellow Bridge which would get you back to where you began. This was about 3 miles and we did it in 45 to 50 minutes every day at lunch. That's 15 miles a week! It was **fun** AND **simple**.

Granted, not everyone can have this kind of walk (*I was lucky to have it for about 6 months*). But, in most towns or cities, there is something that you can do that is pretty good. You need to keep it fairly **close to work or home** so you can start it quickly without much effort.

Exercise such as this will tone you and help you improve your cardiovascular health. It will burn calories and increase your metabolism.

This way of getting exercise is both EFFECTIVE and EASY. This is by design. As with the food aspect of the Weight Loss In Steps system, it's critical that **the exercise is palatable**. If you get to the point where you dread it, you won't be apt to keep it up.

Fortunately, more and more people are beginning to realize that you don't have to kill yourself with exercise to get tremendous benefit from it. **Walking is a perfect choice**.

The Dials

The more steps you take the more this system will be able to work for you. This is the case for the dials too. The more dials you use and turn up, the more this system will be able to work for you!

PROTEIN Dial

Have three 2 to 3 ounce portions of these kinds of protein a day: **white fish, chicken, turkey, egg white**.

Adding another 2 or 3 servings of a high-quality **whey** protein is ok. This is optional.

Don't have red meat and any meat with salt added.

CARB Dial

Eliminate white flour, white rice/pasta and white potato.

This can be very hard for some people to do. Here is one way to slowly take this on:

- Start having no white carb **meals**.
- Then start having no white carb **days**.
- Then start having no white carb **weeks**.

Don't beat yourself up for not being able to do this cold turkey. White carb food tastes delicious. It's normal to want it.

What I have found is, *if I give myself this kind of control*, I am not apt to crave it a lot and binge.

Over time, I really find myself **naturally and happily** having no white carb days and sometimes even no white carb weeks. It has taken years for me to get to this point.

The good news is, you notice your body responding well **even** when you **slowly reduce** your white carb intake.

MEALS Dial

Break your food consumption into 5 to 6 mini meals a day. **This stokes your metabolism**. And, make sure you start eating fairly early in the morning and finish before it gets late at night.

Specifically, have your first meal of the day by **8 AM**. And have your last meal of the day by **8 PM**.

Eating something about every two hours is ideal. Make sure you have a protein portion for breakfast, lunch and dinner.

SALT Dial

For some of you even low salt eating may not be quite enough. NO salt eating is not as bad as it sounds. You definitely need to make sure you **have some key ingredients** on hand. The Mrs. Dash products help enormously here. So does lemon and various vinegars. And always be on the look out for more. For example, I have recently found that fresh parsley is helpful.

Not having any salt still can be very hard for some people to do. Here is one way to slowly take this on:

- Start having **no salt** individual **meals**. They do add up!
- Then start having **no salt days**.

Salt is an incredibly powerful and effective flavor enhancer. So, it shouldn't come as a surprise that this is another one of those areas that takes time to embrace.

But, the fact that you have full control seems to give you the courage to stick with it, even if it's only a meal at a time, every now and again. Seeing really positive results from this can also give you the motivation to be persistent even if you aren't doing a lot with it.

 It is actually kind of fun to figure out how to construct a meal that tastes delicious without salt. Almost anyone can make a good tasting meal with salt. It's definitely a challenge to make a good tasting meal without it. But, **it is possible** to do.

A **salt-sensitive body** will thank you over and over again for working with this dial.

BEVERAGES Dial

Eliminate alcohol, caffeine, and soda.

This can be very hard to do, especially for all of these. Here is one way to slowly take this on:

- Start having **no bad beverages meals**.
- Then start having **no bad beverages days**.

Periodic no bad beverage consumption such as this, will help your body over time.

Some among us can/want to eliminate all bad beverages indefinitely. Many of you (including me) will not be completely eliminating these beverages. Know that **even** mindful **reduction** here and there **helps** your body.

I have found that switching from coffee to green tea is a great first step in terms of minimizing the caffeine aspect. Because of the benefits of green tea, many of you may want to stop there (and have 1 – 3 cups of green tea a day).

Others may eventually feel you are ready to move on from that. Assuming you still want warm beverages throughout the day, especially during cooler times of the year, I'd recommend that you start to drink herbal teas. They have evolved considerably over the last few decades. I am a big fan of herb teas with chamomile and ginger in them. There are probably hundreds of kinds to choose from today. Have fun!

This Isn't The End!

If you'd like to share how you are doing with this way of eating, please feel free to post your feedback on Facebook: http://www.facebook.com/weightlossinsteps

All feedback is carefully reviewed & may be used to evolve this material!

A Weight Loss In Steps recipe book is in the works too!